# SILENT VOICES

# SILENT VOICES

## A Mother's & Teacher's Perspective Of Autism

SUZY DELL

XULON PRESS

Xulon Press
2301 Lucien Way #415
Maitland, FL 32751
407.339.4217
www.xulonpress.com

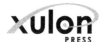

Unless otherwise indicated, Scripture quotations taken from the King
James Version (KJV) – *public domain.*

Paperback ISBN-13: 978-1-6628-2459-3
Ebook ISBN-13: 978-1-6628-2460-9

# Chapter one

My first child was born in November of 1992, a beautiful, angel-faced, petite girl named Maddi. All of my friends had little boys and when they would look at her, they said she looked like a perfect, little baby doll with an angelic face. Of course, I was so proud to hear how pretty they thought she was in her little cradle, made for her by her grandfather.

My son was born on a turbulent afternoon in April of 1994. This was when my adult struggles as a Christian educator, mother, and wife began. You see, I was married at age twenty-four, fairly young considering today's modern standards. I met my husband Phil in 1988, dated him one year, and we were married in June of 1989. Life seemed perfect in so many ways. I began my career as a secondary teacher in Texas in August of 1989 and it became an extraordinary learning year. My first year to teach was in a small town in Texas, which was where I went to school my entire life and graduated in 1983. In a town of 4,000, I had many long-time friends and family there, and it was great to start my career where I had grown up as a child.

I had wonderful, Christian parents and, for the most part, a largely biblical community. I was reared in Texas, also known as the Bible Belt. My idea of life was somewhat naïve and limited growing up. Although my parents were both believers, my mom was the leading spiritual person in our household. My dad did not attend church very often until he was elderly and sick with colon cancer.

This would be my strong, spiritual roots growing into a large strong oak, as life progressed with branches representing my choices and challenges. I wanted to write this memoir with the hope that I may pass spiritual wisdom, educational insight, and parental guidance to others as to what worked best for me on this spiritual, educational journey of mine into autism. Thirty-one years in education, thirty-one years in a marriage, and twenty-seven years as a parent of two awesome, adult children. I hope to give young parents a hope for a bright, spiritual journey with their special needs children, as well as their siblings.

First, I would like to express my amazement and awe at how Jesus has been with me, my family, my students, and the many communities I have had the privilege of teaching and living in over the years. I believe this journey was laid out before the foundations of the earth and is God-directed every step of the way, in spite of the agony of some of my experiences and circumstances along the way.

After my husband Phil and I married in 1989, we both jumped head first into long careers as a chemist and teacher, respectively. My husband and I started as total opposites in a lot of ways, and as I was to discover, this was both a blessing and a curse in so many ways. Besides the fact that Phil seemed totally left brained and I seemed totally right brained, there were many other issues that would spring to the surface as time went on in our marriage. I would venture to say this is something most marriages experience.

You see, there were times in my life when I was very close to Jesus and other times, I was running away from Him. Whether it was fear or rebellion, I'm sure the spiritual forces were fighting one another daily and moment to moment. Some of these memories are burned into my brain like a hot iron, to where people tell me they are amazed at how much I can remember.

Growing up in a small town with Christian parents in a Christian community, for the most part, is something that I praise God for every day. This environment was the seed or foundation, if you will, that would help me to continue my Christian faith no matter what came my way. Many times, the armor of God was protecting me. Even when I couldn't feel it or see it, I had the shield of faith. This faith would grow stronger and stronger as I grew older, because sometimes that little seed beginning was my oak and all I could hold onto. To my utter amazement, Jesus would show up and show off in ways I hadn't planned or imagined.

My first three years of marriage were rather smooth, as Phil and I settled into our home and careers. These were our only two focuses at the time. I was spiritually up and down at this point because I began to realize my husband and I had different ideas about life. He and I traveled these first three years. When I say traveled, it was within our budget; within the United States in a car. We took so many pictures, visited relatives from all walks of life, and marveled at how well our careers and our relationship were going.

Now looking back, I see I always loved the Lord but didn't always put Him first, love Him, and serve Him as I should have. Sometimes, to my amazement, He used me when I didn't even know He had until I looked back and remember it. So perspective, attitude, and belief in Jesus is everything. I was weak, but He was strong.

After two years of mostly a blissful marriage, getting to know one another, and becoming friends, we moved into a townhouse in The woodlands, Texas from where we were living in Beaumont, Texas. Phil and I both had grown up in Texas. Phil had grown up in a strict but loving Catholic family in Beaumont, where mass was required. He was the fourth of five children. I often heard stories of their childhood from his three sisters and one brother. They were very similar yet different in many ways from my own. God definitely had a plan for Phil and I, and this was just one example that seemed more than coincidence.

My mom and my mother-in-law were in the same hospital, on the same week in the same year. My mother was in the Baptist hospital in Beaumont, Texas, giving birth to her second child, Suzy (me), and then my mom-in-law checked in five days later to give birth to my sister-in-law Paige. I never realized this until a few years back when my husband pointed it out. Detail is his thing being a scientist. I believe this was the first of many proofs of how Jesus is so involved in our lives. He loves us with an unending and unconditional love that we can't even imagine or perceive, always pointing us in His righteous way.

I was reared in the Methodist church where my mother brought my brothers and me frequently. Every summer, she dropped us off there for Vacation Bible School, where we had wonderful people who did their best to love us, teach us, and entertain us until Mom arrived to pick us up. My husband attended every Vacation Bible School that was offered in Beaumont at every church his mom could find. With five children, I'm sure this was a great and needed escape.

My mom and Phil's mom taught us early about the Bible, church, and community. When Phil and I married in 1989, it was in the Methodist church that was so dear to my heart because I was reared there. Phil said he was not interested in jumping through all of Catholic counseling and hoops of the Catholic Church. He said the Methodist church will work.

# CHAPTER TWO

# Our Blessed Hope–New Life

———

My story is one of hope, fear, persistence, and testing because I also believe as the Bible teaches that trials and tests are big parts of our journey. Little did I know this background of faith would be so needed in the years following our wedding. Shortly after moving to The Woodlands, Texas, my husband and I decided to embark on a new adventure of buying our first home. We didn't have a lot of money at the time, so we saved and found a hungry realtor named Tom to help us find our perfect starter home. Just like I did in 1989, with getting married and starting a career, I was ready to add two more branches to our oak tree: buying a home and starting a family. I was six weeks pregnant when we moved into our first home. Our friends Traci and Mikey helped us move in. Thank you Jesus for sending Your help.

My firstborn, Madison, was born in November very close to Thanksgiving, two weeks early to our surprise. I went to my regularly scheduled doctor's appointment with Dr. Winter two weeks before my estimated due date. Little did I know when driving to Dr. Winter's office that I would embark on another journey, beginning with a trial. I never left my appointment. The nurse's eyes got wide, after taking my initial blood pressure, and said, "I'm going to get the doctor."

This was my first child, so what was going on? Fear began to set in. Dr. Winter arrived in the tiny exam room and began taking my blood pressure after the nurse had already done so. This was irritating and frightening. He took the pressure, then he told me I couldn't go home. I was like, "What and why? What's going on?" He said, "Just walk over to Memorial Hospital next door." Again, naïvely not knowing that once I entered the hospital, the struggle to have my firstborn would begin.

Before leaving the doctor's office, I had to alert my husband at work about what was going on. Back in the early nineties, there were no cellphones. Can you imagine? When he answered his lab phone, I calmly told him to meet me at the hospital, saying, "Doctor said I had to go." Phil is my rock so I'm sure he kept it together on his way there, which was only a ten minute-drive from his work in the Woodlands. Upon arrival, nurses had me laying down, started an IV, and were monitoring blood pressure.

Shortly after Phil arrived, he was given the task of contacting my parents. My dad was working in one of the refineries as a pipefitter in Port Arthur at the time. He was called off the job by my mom, Polly. We were informed shortly after arriving that I would be induced because of my high blood pressure, a condition called Toxemia or Preeclampsia. I had been on bed rest for two weeks and my mom had stayed with me and cooked healthy food for me, but it didn't work. There I was a week later in the hospital with extremely high blood pressure.

So I was induced the next morning and placed in intensive care. At first, it didn't work, so after several hours of my family coming into intensive care, one by one, the nurse kicked them all out and said for me to choose just one person to come in. Sorry Phil, I chose my Dad; I really didn't want to look at the person who had started this whole thing. Anyway, my Dad, Maurice, just sat next to me quietly and held my hand. Of course, Phil was my rock, but at the time my Dad was too. I felt like a little girl who needed her Daddy.

After sitting with me for a long time, I ordered him, my mom, mother-in-law, and Phil's Aunt Norma and Uncle Bob to go home and rest. I told them I was fine, so They left to eat and rest. As soon as I relaxed because I was alone and it was quiet, my water broke. I panicked; oh no, I just sent my family home so I had the nurse call them all to come back. They came back immediately, not wanting to miss their first child and grandchild being born. Little did I know that, again, I had a new trial as I would now be in labor for sixteen hours and be clinging to my intensive care nurse. This was another "Jesus lives" moment, as He was with me way more than I knew. My daughter, who was born that night; and is now 27 years old is an intensive care nurse at our local hospital.

After sixteen hours of excruciating labor, the doctor arrived in full scrub wear, asking me if I knew what this meant. He had on the blue scrubs, so I naturally said, "Is it a boy?" Everyone began laughing and said, "No, it's time for a C-section." I told them I wanted to remain awake for the birth of my daughter so I stayed awake during the surgery to see her arrival at 6 lbs., 11 oz. She was beautiful and I will never forget the looks of pure joy, pride, and peace on my husband's face when she was born. We had a year and seventeen months of bliss with our first child Maddi.

I grew closer to Jesus, knowing that He was the beginning and the end, and He works all things for the good for those of us who love Him. Maddi reached all her milestones early and began to walk at eight months old while her Dad was away in Germany working. I didn't want to travel with him out of the United States. He was so sad he didn't see her first steps, but a manager told him he most likely would have been at work when it happened even if he were working in the US. My husband's career had really taken off at this point, and he was now working for Hewlett Packard as a scientist: higher salary, greater benefits, but more time away from his family. Everything comes with a price, and this took a toll on our marriage.

Two weeks later, when he arrived home, let's just say he was happy to see us, and I became pregnant again. As I sat on the couch and cried, he and Madison danced around the house in excitement when the pregnancy test was positive. I remember calling my sister-in-law Paige to tell her I was pregnant again. She screamed; I think she was in shock because her children were more spread out age-wise. I was a little scared because of what occurred in my first pregnancy.

# CHAPTER THREE

## Arrival Of Jordan On A Stormy Day

———

My son Jordan was born on a turbulent, stormy afternoon in April. Little did I know again of the storms ahead. I ate healthy and exercised through both pregnancies, but I came to learn through talking with my mom that I had a great aunt, Georgia, who died in childbirth. She had the same condition as me, where she never dilated. My grandmother testified to everyone that an angel came to her the night of her sister's horrific labor to tell her and her mother to go to Georgia. Because she died in the early 1900s from this condition, I know what a medical and spiritual miracle had occurred during my daughter's birth, and that same miracle was scheduled to happen again.

I was checked into the hospital again two weeks early with Toxemia. I would not have to suffer as much with this pregnancy, since the doctor just scheduled the C-section this time. I stayed awake for this C-section as well, even though the doctors tried to talk me out of doing this. They said I would feel more because of this being my second C-section, but I defiantly told them no. I would not be put to sleep; I want to witness my baby being born. The doctors said no more, since I had made my decision.

I stared out the hospital window and noticed the darkening sky. I believe this sky was foreshadowing our lives to come. I was calm this time, as I knew what was going to take place. Everything went fairly smooth, except when I required some oxygen. Before we knew it, we were holding an awesome baby boy! Thank you, Jesus, for my two miracles! My dad kept telling Phil what a fine boy we had. He was so excited to have another grandchild.

# CHAPTER FOUR

# The Colors Of Life

———

The first couple of years with Jordan were quite normal. It was only hectic because I had two small children in diapers and a double stroller at once. People would say, "Look, she has two babies." My kids were so close in age that it seemed like they were twins sometimes. However, this story is a story of fear, hope, persistence, and one of the greatest tests a family can endure. Phil and I had plans to become parents again. We discussed having more children, but when Jordan was two, my husband said that was good having just two children and scheduled his vasectomy.

My earliest recollection of our family crisis was when Jordan turned three years old. We had a big birthday party at a park in Tyler, Texas, where we had recently built a home; a beautiful, ranch-style home with big front and back porches. We gave our builder our blueprints, and he loved the style we chose and later referred customers to the floor plan. I remember building a home as such a blessing! We put our children's handprints on the back porch concrete as a way to say home sweet home. But as they say, men make plans, and God laughs.

At Jordan's birthday party, we invited family and friends. Our builder and his wife Vanessa showed up to give Jordan this awesome computer game. Mark and Vanessa explained that their 3-year-old Kate had a rare disorder that had caused her to have brain damage. Mark and Vanessa were fellow church members at our church. I remember the absolute despair they described to us as they received her diagnosis, their questioning God as to why would this happen. They thought somehow this was their fault and even wondered if God was punishing them for something. I quickly told them that Jesus wasn't punishing them, what a blessing their daughter was, and how sickness and disease come from Satan. God had not done this to her.

I thought back to Adam and Eve and their original sin that brought sickness and disease to the world. I had met people who said they couldn't believe in a God that would allow such a thing as sickness to happen. I remember thinking, *No, it's just the world we live in; God doesn't want to hurt or harm us.* Before this third birthday party began, we were so happy, sending invitations and buying balloons, gifts, and burgers to cook. We never saw this coming, this mountainous blow our family was about to take.

The next day, Jordan's birthday arrived with much anticipation and excitement. Phil took out our video camera, which by the way was one of the first ones made; a dinosaur by today's standards. We were excited to capture the entire event on tape. Now I know how much our family would later need that tape to bring ourselves out of denial and into reality.

Jordan's party started as any party would, with the opening of lots of presents. As we handed him each gift, he didn't even want to try to open them! Strange but whatever; we thought he was just shy. He just sat there and stared into space. My husband tried desperately to get his attention, but this only agitated Jordan and he began to kick and scream loudly and uncontrollably. I wondered if my husband had been this way as a child. My mother-in-law didn't say anything, while I tried to explain his tantrum behavior away. I didn't remember my daughter throwing these explosive, loud tantrums. As I recall, she played, sang, ran, opened gifts, ate cake, and spoke with the utmost excitement for her party.

My motherly instinct kicked in, saying to myself, *Why are you comparing your children? They are very different. Jordan is just quiet like his Daddy, unless he doesn't get what he wants. This is just his personality.* As I thought about what I had just thought and remembered, a small dose of panic entered my brain. *What if something is wrong? On second thought, Jordan doesn't even play with toys, or even other children for that matter; no interaction. That's it! An epiphany; he just needs some socialization. Phil, Madison, and I alone must not be meeting all of his socialization needs. I will call the church on Monday, and maybe he can go to the Mother's Day Out program at our church. Yes, that's all he needs!*

As the party came to an end, my mom and my mother-in-law lingered. My brother-in-law Dillon, who was a local elementary principal, made a statement at Jordan's party that was really bothering me. Dillion asked us if Jordan was talking yet. *What a strange question*, I thought. Well, no, he really isn't but I wasn't worried; after all, he was a quiet, shy boy. However, I could tell at the end of the party that my mom had something on her mind. My mom wouldn't be able to contain her thoughts. She was known for speaking her mind on occasion; otherwise, she was always very courteous and sweet. My mother-in-law kept quiet; she didn't give any advice unless asked, or at least that is what she tried to do in this case.

My mom began to question Jordan's tantrum, odd behaviors, and lack of speech. He didn't play with his toys like other kids she remarked. *She is right*, I thought. *He lines up his cars rather than driving them around. That is different. Oh well, sometimes you get a different child.* Now, I am thankful for my outspoken brother-in-law and mother.

Ok, so my mom was thinking along the same lines as me; time for questioning my in-laws about my husband's behavior as a child. I will get to the bottom of this, or so I thought. My mom reminisced about babysitting Jordan at her home , while I was working as a teacher, and we were busy building our new home. We lived with our mom and dad while we were building our home in another small Texas town, which was, for the most part, a good experience. After my mother had voiced her concerns, my mother- in-law, Debby, chimed in. This was her chance to verbalize her opinion. Granny Debby commented that Phil had talked at Jordan's age.

Ok so this led to me questioning my sister-in-law Sharon. I asked her, "Did Katy (her youngest child) talk at age three?" Yes, I was trying to convince myself that maybe his nonverbal behavior was just some family trait. "No," Sharon replied. "Katy talked at two." Then I quickly asked another question. "Was Katy a quiet child? I don't remember her talking much." "Was Katy a quiet child?" Sharon replied. "Yes, a quiet child." Now confusion was setting in. I know who spreads confusion, the enemy. Then, with this last question, all the family guests began to scurry home. I questioned myself for questioning them. *Did my Mom and I make them feel uncomfortable in some way?*

Probably all of our questions, my husband's family seemed like very private people compared to my family. *Ok*, I thought to myself, *my Mom and I are just worry warts!* Then when the in-laws had departed, it was just my Mom and me sitting there quietly lost in our thoughts. But my Mom wasn't letting this go. She said, "Suzy, don't you think Jordan should be talking by now?" What was this, an intervention or something? Why is everyone so concerned about my baby? *Now she was getting under my skin a little. I think it is time for her to go home too,* I thought to myself. "No, Mom," I quickly retorted. "Jordan is just a quiet child like his father and his family. Phil doesn't talk often either." I then declared, "Jordan will talk when he is ready," thinking there was nothing wrong with my perfect, little boy. Even then, I remember my Mom was not convinced. She pushed me again and just wouldn't let it go.

I was thirty-one years old at the time and I remember thinking, *This is just how all Moms are when they know something just isn't quite right.* My Mom thought I should call Jordan's pediatrician on Monday, Dr. Lerrick. I argued with her a little, then conceded to call him because her final words seared my heart. She said, "If there isn't anything wrong, what does it hurt just to have a check-up?" Well, that sounded very reasonable and I had been convinced. I wanted to quickly put this to rest. But little did I know this was going to be a marathon in my life, not a sprint.

That night, as things were winding down from the party, I remembered I needed to check my answering machine. This answering machine was awesome in the eighties and nineties.

Anyway, I don't remember how many messages I listened to but one particular one resonates with me. I will get to the message shortly, but looking back, it was a message from Jesus trying His best to help me using my friend (and fellow Christian) Tiffany. Tiffany and I met shortly after I met her husband and his buddy, Phil.

I met Phil and Jerry at the locate dance hot spot, the Sunny Club, at the hotel in Tyler, Texas. That night is forever etched in my brain as I know God spoke to me that night, telling me to give my now-husband a chance. My instinct was to write him off at first that night, but that's when God spoke to me about Phil. It was a thought that came into my head that night when I tried to brush Phil off. I was thinking he was just like the rest of the guys I've met, where he would take my number and most likely not call. You see, Jerry asked me to dance first. I gave him one look and decided, No, I don't want to dance, as I stood there being snobby to someone who would be my future friend. Later, I found out my to be dear friend Tiffany was Jerry's girlfriend at the time he was out dancing. I guess Tiffany was at home waiting for him. Jerry finally got to dance with me at he and Tiffany's daughter's wedding. Funny how things happen!

As I stood alone, this tall, dark-haired, good-looking guy came over to me and asked me if I wanted to dance. I gave him one look and said, "Yes." We took off dancing and, wow, he could dance. We were fast dancing. After several dances, he asked me for my phone number. I told him no as nicely as I could and began to walk away.

I stopped dead in my tracks just a few seconds away when I heard this voice speak to me that I now know was God trying to order my steps. The thought or voice of God said simply, "Well, maybe he is a nice guy, not like the rest." Well, the Bible says as Christians we know the voice of our Good Shepherd. *Hmm,* I thought, *maybe he is.* I complied with the thought (silent voice) and quickly turned around in my tracks. So that was it; we were married a year later. Phil at twenty-five years old and me at twenty-four years old. Not knowing what the years would have in store for us, we jumped in head-first.

Back to my friend Tiffany: So she left a message on Jordan's third birthday, asking if everything was ok with us. *That was strange,* I thought, as I called her back and told her everything was fine. No problems here, everything is great! She said, "Well, God laid you and Phil on my heart. I've had a burden and I've been praying for you guys." I thought to myself, *a burden, a burden about what?*

# CHAPTER FIVE

# The Long Spiritual Road

---

W hen Monday arrived, I called Dr. Lerrick's office and made an appointment for Jordan's check-up. I dressed Jordan and waited for my mom Polly to arrive to babysit Madison. I needed my mom to help with her, because I knew she needed love, care, and attention. My mom was there to provide. Thank you, Jesus! My brain began to tell me that I was just overreacting as usual. *Yes, I'm overreacting, Dr. Lerrick will put this question to rest and Jordan will be just fine.*

As soon as I arrived at Dr. Lerrick's office, Jordan began to leap from my arms and run around the office wildly. He hid under the chairs and tables and made strange noises. The other mothers began to stare at us, making me feel as if they were judging me because I had no control over this child. Maybe I did, maybe I didn't. I judged myself as I tried my best to settle him down, chasing him around. Phil's sisters had told me stories of how bad Jordan's dad had been as a child. I thought, *Well, maybe he just had ADHD or something.* No one really diagnosed it very well during the sixties and seventies. Somehow, those funny stories about Phil weren't so funny anymore.

The office wait seemed everlasting, as I continued to chase Jordan around this small waiting room. I tried in vain to get him to be seated quietly like the other children. Now the nurses and office workers were beginning to stare at Jordan and I. *This is odd,*

I thought. *Why is my child the only one who won't sit down? What is wrong with me? Nothing,* I rationalized. *He is just a boy.*

Finally, Jordan's name was called. Thank God, I was exhausted trying to contain him. Dr. Lerrick quickly came to the room; obviously, this mother and child had been reported to him. I began the process of explaining the situation. All of a sudden, his face looked so sad. After his initial look of pity, he stated that Jordan would immediately need some speech therapy. Alright, no problem, my own younger brother had needed that in school. No big deal. Dr. Lerrick hurried off to call E.C.I. (Early Childhood Intervention). *Who is E.C.I.?* I thought as he left the room to call them.

He returned rather quickly to tell me that because Jordan had recently turned three years old that he no longer qualified for free speech services. OK, now what? Just great, this was very upsetting. He suggested we visit a local speech therapist at her clinic. I then proceeded to tell the doctor that Jordan had been in a local church's Mother's Day Out program. He thought that was a great idea, except I said the caretakers at the church nursery had suggested that I get Jordan's ears tested. I explained to them that Jordan could hear fine. I know when I make a noise, such as rolling a toy truck, he turned his head.

After suggesting that Jordan have his hearing checked, his teacher said he had repeated the word Jesus once while she was changing his diaper and singing to him. She pointed at Jesus's picture above the changing table and he had said, "Jesus." Wow! Was this his first word at age three? I decided that I would observe Jordan in his Mother's Day Out to see if he interacted with any other children. As I watched Jordan, he sat in a corner of the room, sucking his thumb, then lying down and rolling around on the floor. I quickly picked him up and put him with the other children. He went straight back to the corner to suck his thumb and roll around. This was disheartening.

Back to Dr. Lerrick's office and our conversation about Jordan's ears. Dr. Lerrick concluded that testing Jordan's ears would be another step in the testing process. *Testing? Testing for what?* All of a sudden, the word "autistic" popped into my head. *Could this be what he is testing for?* Even though the word had leaped into my thoughts during the observation at Mother's Day Out, I was still clearly in some form of denial. Dr. Lerrick agreed that checking his hearing also wasn't a bad idea, so he also referred us to a local audiologist, Dr. Henry, for testing. I would get an appointment there first.

The very next day, I took Jordan to the audiologist, who found no hearing problem or hearing loss . I already knew that would be the outcome somehow. I looked directly into Dr. Henry's eyes and asked her directly, "What would cause my child not to speak, if it isn't a hearing problem?" She gave me that all too familiar look of pity. Then there was this melancholy silence again between us. The word "autistic" came back into my mind. What did I know about Autism? I had only observed it once on *60 Minutes* and I was saddened by watching the children rocking back and forth, saying nothing or making strange noises.

Then seeing the concern, and maybe even a little panic in my face, she said, "I just tested a baby with teenage parents that had a child that was born with his intestines on the outside of his body." She then said, "They are doing just fine with the baby." Oh my gosh, *What was she trying to say? I should feel blessed because it could always be worse?* I guess she was right. Well, one thing was for sure; Jordan could hear but he had only spoken the name of Jesus once. What a first word, just couldn't get it out of him again.

Yes, you didn't have to tell me how blessed I was with two healthy children. I had a grandfather with one leg, he swore he had lost his ear in a fight with an old bear at a circus during the Great Depression. He said he won $5 dollars which was a whole lot of money in those days. I think that was why he was missing one ear. I had heard stories of my great- grandmother, Ma Dell, making him do not doing everything all of the other children did, then she would go to her room to cry. She didn't want her six children, J.J. being the oldest, to see her cry, even though her husband, Johnney Waylon, had left her for some other woman during the Depression with six children to rear alone.

My Pa Pa J.J., being the oldest, didn't finish high school because he went to work to support his mother and five younger siblings.

I also heard stories of my Ma Dell going to bed every night not eating, or eating as little as possible, so she could feed her children. I remember her being a tall, thin woman. She made the best tea cups (cookies) and hot-water cornbread you have ever tasted in your life. I still make her hot-water cornbread for my husband to go with Granny Dell's homemade vegetable beef soup.

I had another childhood experience with a disability known as Spina Bifida. My first cousin was born with it and was one of the Lathi Amide baby. These were the babies born in the early sixties whose mothers were given a lathi amide pill for their nausea, not knowing it would cause their children to be born with an open spine. My first cousin, Waylon, was born and they said my Grandma Dell passed out at the hospital when she learned the news that her first grandchild was born with spina bifida. My aunt and uncle went on to have two healthy girls after Waylon.

But soon after they were born, my aunt divorced my uncle, because of lots of things I'm sure of. But one thing I am sure of is my aunt and uncle had the odds against them because 75 percent of couples who have a disabled child divorce, as opposed to 50 percent of couples with non-disabled children. Okay, so this was some family background, and I had some experience with disabilities. I also had some experiences with perseverance and boy, would I need it in the years to come.

My cousin was treated as normal as possible. The doctors operated on him hundreds of times before my aunt and uncle's divorce around his age of five. Waylon lived his life in a wheelchair and was no stranger to pain, but he drove a car with hand controls, graduated from a university with a bachelor's degree, worked as a dispatch in a sheriff's department, volunteered at a United Way program in Tyler, Texas, and lived to be fifty, defying all the doctor's predictions and odds. Did I mention he never missed a football game at his school or his mother's school? My aunt was a school counselor. This helped Waylon tremendously, as you might imagine.

Within a few days, Phil, Jordan, and I proceeded to our next testing stop: the speech therapist's office. Melody came out with a large, bright, noisy rain-stick in her hand. Wow, this got everyone's attention, especially Jordan's. We observed her as she caught Jordan's attention, and worked and worked with Jordan, and then finally a word! He repeated a word that she asked him to say. It was "POP." In his excitement, he repeated this word each time he popped the bubbles she blew into the air. You see, I was in denial. I thought, *Jordan can talk when he wants to talk*.

After this expensive session, I quickly asked the therapist what would cause Jordan not to talk. Again, that pity stare and silence, then she held out a business card to my husband Phil and I. It read Dr. Woodson, Ph.D. (child psychologist). Fear and panic immediately set in. Jordan is Autistic. They think Jordan is Autistic. Autism was first coined by Leo Kanner in 1943, who defined it as a severe disorder of thinking, communication, interpersonal relationships, and behavior. I had learned this definition as a Pedagogy major in college, but never thought I would encounter it, especially not in my own child!

# CHAPTER SIX

## Denial And Despair Set In

---

I t seemed the denial stage of the Autism diagnosis in our family was going to be crashing down as quickly as it came with a diagnosis for Jordan. Those early days were only the beginning of a long, hard, and frustrating journey for my family and I. This tragedy definitely turned into triumph in many ways along our journey. When Jordan was three, following his diagnosis from the psychologist, Dr. Woodson, Phil and I sprang into action. We immediately contacted our local university, Lamar University, with our applied behavior analysis report and plan and diagnosis. I quickly made my way to the educational department there. *A special education professor is what we needed,* I concluded.

Upon visiting Dr. Goudas, she agreed to send special education students out to our home in Tyler to implement the first applied behavior program in the area. Phil and I had done our research and we naively thought that this would somehow fix or cure Jordan. It helped Jordan tremendously, but there was no cure. During this time, from three to nine years old, we taught Jordan at home, in preschool, and into elementary school. During these years, we continued to try to cure or help our son.

All the while, my little girl Madison was excelling in her elementary school and was placed in the gifted and talented program there. My Mom and Mother- in-law rushed into help me, as I rushed Jordan and Madison from one appointment to another.

My husband provided for us and underwent his own frustration. He began traveling more and more it seemed. It was great for the pay, but I felt I needed a lot more than his pay. He and I needed each other and needed to continue this journey together. We read books at night together in bed, and I prayed like I have never prayed before. One night, I felt I literally had a severe panic attack. I got in my bathtub and cried and cried until I got in bed to cry and cry more. Phil did the best he could to help me through my depression, even though he had his own depression and challenges to deal with.

I never stopped teaching Madison and Jordan, and my students at the Taylor Career Center where I was a high school English teacher. When Phil and I were first married, I taught English in high schools and junior high schools during this time. I would eventually retire from the public school system at Port Arthur where I taught at the Motiva Youth Training Academy as a business teacher. After and in between my teaching in the public school system, I also taught at two private Christian schools, a charter school, and at Partners Resource Network funded by the Department of Education. There I worked two years as a parent advocate for parents of children with special needs. I even got to travel to Austin with my boss and attend a T.E.A. (Texas Education Agency) board meeting. This was very helpful and informative in understanding the school system, especially for children with disabilities.

During the same time, I was teaching and my husband was working long hours, I fell into a depression, as Jordan was having more and more tantrums during the next few years. I began to start my own business, as well, to help parents advocate for their children's programs in schools. I attended ARDS (admission, review, and dismissal) meetings in public school with other parents, discovering that this was a huge problem for lots of people who had a lot less education and resources than I did, so I went into this helping parents discover their rights stage. During this time, my daughter was ten and my son was nine, and I wrote to express my feelings during this time period.

I was published in the International Library of Poetry in the volume "Colors of Life." The poem was an expression of my feelings at the time, which I felt were very important to document all of these feelings along the way. This is my poem:

Autism emerges, night plunges to grief, day awakens us, questions originate, answers impel, walls form, hope is deferred, false hope, the clock ticks, hopelessness awaits, new beginnings, small miracles come, acceptance, happiness, growth dawns.

My dad would not read it when I told him what my poem was about. You see, this disability, as all disabilities, affects everyone in the family in one way or another. Hopefully, and prayerfully, it affects you more positively than negatively. Writing was part of my therapy, while the Scripture, Romans 8:28, that all things work for the good for those who love God and who are called for His purpose certainly applies to my life. The Scripture also of Jeremiah 29:11, "I know the plans I have for you, plans to help you and not hurt you, says the Lord" helps too. The Scriptures encouraged me during these difficult times where time would not stop to give me a break. How I had wished to stop the clock from ticking. Valuable time with my children was slipping away.

During the years, from three to nine years old, we tried the Applied Behavioral Analysis(ABA), TEEACH & PECS schedules, vitamin supplements and enzymes, specific glutton and sugarfee, and additive diet programs, speech, occupational therapy, swimming with sign language, music, assistive technology, and the list goes on. In our desperation, we tried some experimental trials of hormones and sought an allergist to help us with supplements and hormones. This allergist explained to us that he wasn't Jesus Christ of Nazareth. He was trying not to give us false hope.

The psychologist Dr. Woodson explained that every few years or so someone was offering some miracle cure. We wanted a miracle! I prayed for one and went to church believing that this would go away somehow. These treatments were expensive, and Jordan's grandparents helped us pay. We traveled back and forth to Dallas, I guess, still trying to fix Jordan. My dad would tell me that he would fix it for me if he could. He was such a loving example of how I saw my Father in heaven, who wanted to assist us in our needs.

Jordan went through the public school system, while his sister was put into private school, then public school. What a blessing the Christian schools were to her and I at this time. She excelled in everything. Madison and Jordan were high achievers, only in different ways and styles. They both could sing beautifully. Madison sang "Happy Birthday Jesus" in her public school elementary one Christmas to a standing ovation. She and Jordan got their voices from their dad, as Phil is musically talented.

At seven, we began taking Jordan to a psychiatrist in the Beaumont, Texas area, who I quickly became friends with. She was affectionately known as Dr. Cupcakes. She was a huge help in the next few years to come, not only with medications to ease Jordan's symptoms of anxiety but with suggestions for programs for Jordan; not to mention she also addressed my depression. She explained to me that needing medication for an anxiety disorder like I have that leads to panic disorder is not a sign of weakness in anyway. This statement helped me to begin to treat my depression. She was a Christian and I know Jesus sent Jordan and I to her. She was part of God's good plan for our lives.

# CHAPTER SEVEN

# Depart From Me, You Wicked Principalities In High Places

---

Ten years later, when Madison was thirteen and Jordan was twelve, we decided to depart from the school district. We had been battling them for years to try and get them to help our son in a way we felt he needed and deserved. I studied the special education laws and knew what was best for him as his mom. Besides the fact, my daughter was a social butterfly and was exceling in school. Jordan was not excelling and was plunging into and banging his head against metal poles. It was horrific. He was coming home with bruises on his forehead where he was banging his head. I took a picture in my horror, but later threw the picture away because I didn't want to ever see it again.

He even began banging his head on our bar where he ate and on our fireplace stones. That was it! Phil and I didn't divorce each other, but we divorced the school district. I wasn't impressed with the special education program or the advanced placement program for my daughter either. Due to a lack of funding, and increasing population in this town, they were getting placed in larger and larger classes. I knew the risk of these large classes, for I had taught in them for myself. Phil and I discussed our options, and fortunately for us, we did have options because of our education, dedication, commitment, resources, and my faith in Jesus.

I put my faith into action quickly, calling on my pastor and fellow church members. I called all the preachers on TBN channel, as well as, emailing Pastor Thyme on TBN. My Mom began to pray like never before, as well as having a feeling a of wanting to run away. Then she fought as a spiritual intercessor does against wicked principalities in high places.

We had several miracles during this time. The first miracle was an answer to my prayers. I was told that I would never convince this school district to help my child in the ways I was asking. They implemented most of the programs I asked them to do, except for the last crucial program I asked of them; that took a special education attorney and a T.E.A. (Texas Education Agency) mediator. Even after all of this, God did answer our prayers for Jordan, and we ended up moving to another school district for the years ahead.

There were two other miracles that occurred during our time in this small town in Texas. My daughter spoke to an angel, and at the age of three years old, described the angels that were guarding our home there. She said they were men angels sitting all over our roof and in our windows. She has no recollection of this, but I woke up to her talking to someone after my panic attack. I asked her who she was talking to, and that is when she told me it was her angel and described all of the angels around our home.

The night before, you see, I had cried out to the Lord to help us the night before with this Autism diagnosis. I had spoken with mothers whose children were sixteen and still in diapers. I was determined not to have the same fate for my son or I. Jordan was out of diapers at five and riding a bike with his sister soon after.

## CHAPTER EIGHT

# More Miracles On The Way

I f the diagnosis of autism and the battles for Jordan's needs weren't enough, my daughter woke up with acute appendicitis at midnight one night. She had not eaten in three days and could barely drink. I had taken her to a doctor three days earlier and he didn't even do bloodwork. She had gone to the school nurse three times that day, asking to go home and the nurse would not let her leave. I was furious. She had never gone to the nurse's office that year, and she was an AP student, so why would she be lying about her pain?

I was tempted to call CPS when they sent my son home with bruises, my daughter home with scratches and scraps from being pushed off the top of monkey bars, and not allowing her to go home when she had a ruptured appendicitis. This school district may have been well meaning for the most part, but now this nurse was definitely negligent. My husband and I brought her to Baptist hospital where Aunt Paige and I were born on the same week. Remember that miracle? How could that have been coincidence? God's so real!

The doctor at the emergency room that night was named Dr. Angie (what an angel). He must have been at the beginning of his career because, later on, I would meet him again as he operated on both of my severe carpal tunnel hands from years of teaching. He later told me that he had twins with Autism. His wife, who was also a doctor, had left her career to care for them. Dr. Angie informed us he believed Madison had acute appendicitis at ten years of age, and he then informed us that the only pediatric surgeon on call was on vacation. I was on the phone at three a.m., speeding back home from Beaumont to get packed and head to Houston's Children's Hospital. My Mother-in-law Debby and her husband Ron came over to care for Jordan.

We rushed our way to the hospital and arrived around six a.m. in the morning, only to be informed that there were critical babies who would go into surgery before her. It was a long and frustrating day, and a long two weeks of lying next to Madison. She left the hospital as a miracle and later would become an R.N. herself after this experience was behind her. She was interested in Cardiology and specialized in this field as a young nurse.

# CHAPTER NINE

# New Beginning And Old Tantrums

My husband and I researched again and found out which school district in the area was the wealthiest. We picked the second wealthiest school district in the area. An excellent school district again, we are the fortunate ones. Some people don't have the means to pick up and leave a town. We were determined, and thank you Jesus for ordering our steps. Jordan and Madison both got the help they needed with very little trouble. No, it wasn't a perfect place, but it definitely was an answer to our many prayers to Jesus and petitions to special education directors.

About a year after settling in there on the coast, we were hit by Hurricane Rita right after Hurricane Katrina. The coastal town we moved to was under a mandatory evacuation order. We left for Stuttgart, Arkansas to spend two weeks with Phil's brother, Jeffrey. We stayed and were fed by the local Methodist church. Delicious Mexican food was on the menu. We were so grateful to have a place to go and food to eat. While we were visiting there, a local Walmart manager, who also had a child with autism, sent us workbooks for free for Jordan to do to keep him busy during this stressful change. Change is very hard for people in general, but especially for children with autism.

When we finally returned to our home on the coast, we found some damage to our home but it was very minimal considering some of our neighbor's homes. Again, I believe God protected us, rescued us, and helped us because we asked Him. After returning home, Jordan, of course, was out of sorts due to all of the recent changes to his schedule. He had started acting out at school again as soon as he returned. Phil traveled, while I struggled to restrain Jordan during tantrums, trying to keep him from hurting himself, his sister, or I. All the while, I was working and cleaning the house and caring for two children. Some days were just too much, and I don't know how people without God cope. He was my everything during this time and now.

I drew closer to God and began to pray again, as Jordan continued to tantrum. He punched holes in our walls and broke some windows. This nightmare was still going. Finally, my mom continued her prayers and visited a sister in Christ to pray with her. She asked my mom one question before she began to pray for her: "What does your daughter want for your grandson?" My mom told her specifically that my daughter wants my grandson to go to a special education school in another town outside of Houston called Mayes Center. It was about three hours north of where we were. The thought of sending him off to school and not seeing him except for some weekends was excruciating, but from all my research I did, this was what he needed.

It was tough love, as my daughter called it, and it felt like it too. Now the only issue was to convince the special education director, who was about to retire, that this needed to be done for Jordan. But how? I quickly tapped into my faith and gave it to Jesus. Only He could fix this problem. How he would do it would be the biggest surprise. He answers our prayers, but not always the way we imagine or think He will.

The next week, my husband took a reprieve from his travels for a couple weeks to be home. Thank God, I thought. I really needed him. I had to call a police officer one night when my husband was gone to help me restrain my son. This was very upsetting. Luckily, I was able to get him restrained right before the officer got there. This was so upsetting to my daughter Maddi, as she was only thirteen years old and loved her brother and was trying to understand all of this chaos that was happening. I held firmly to my faith and prayed.

The next week my husband asked me to sit down on the couch for a minute. He said he needed to talk to me. *Wow, I* thought, *this was scary, with not knowing what he had to say.* He brought out a letter to show me. It was an order from a court concerning my twelve-year-old Jordan. A teacher's paraprofessional was kicked by Jordan in his special education class, and she went to the police and filed charges against him. I was like, "What? Are you serious? How long have you kept this from me?" My husband replied for about a week. He is always trying to protect me, but I immediately flew into action. I called a lawyer first and told him the whole story. He said he couldn't help me and that it was a big mess. I thought, *Well, thanks for nothing*, but God was ordering my steps in this progress. I then wrote a certified letter to the special education director, requesting that she send Jordan to Mayes Achievement Center for his ongoing education.

A long arduous road ahead, it was now somewhat of a blur what happened after Jordan was placed at Mayes Center. I knew he was safe and being well cared for the most part, but the school had formerly been a Baptist church converted to a special education school. What an answer, I hoped, to all of my prayers for God to send angels into our situation. My daughter had seen angels at four years old; now the angels were really involved. She saw them on our roof and I asked her what they looked like. She replied, "Big, strong men, Mommy, and they are in our windows and all over our roof." Wow! I had never seen an angel before. She doesn't remember telling me this in 1996.

This explanation was seared in my brain like a hot iron. Now I was seeing human angels in the men and women at Mayes, who have been working with my son on rules and behavior. This may have been the hardest thing I had to do in my life, leaving my son three hours away with strangers! But this was his only hope in living as normal a life as possible. There was one little boy who was older than Jordan and he had so many behavior problems that he had actually pulled his permanent front teeth out of his mouth. This was extremely disturbing to me; but in the world of Autism, it wouldn't be the first or the last strange Autism symptom I would hear about or know about. All these kids here at Mayes, all the questions whirling in my mind. *How did they get here? What did they do to earn their place here? How long would Jordan be here?*

Then I called Mayes and asked when would be our first visitation with our son. They said we needed to wait thirty days, so we could call him once a week on Sundays or write him as much as we pleased. Oh, my Lord, how we all would cry about this, his dad and I, his sister Maddi, his grandparents, his aunts, his uncles, his cousins. I rushed over to my husband's sister Sharon to tell her what was going on with Jordan's education. Her husband was a principal and would understand what I was going through. Maybe, just maybe, she would give me some words of encouragement to help me make it through. She was a strong woman and would know just what to say to me to help me off this emotional roller coaster!

Surprisingly, she would be silent, then tears ran down her face when I told her we had to place him at Mayes. Then she said, "Could you leave a cell phone with him?" "No" was my answer. She then said, "If it were my children, that that's what I would want to do." Jordan's cousins, Bryan and Katy, were just one year older than Jordan and Maddi; how she must have been empathizing with me!

The night we left Jordan at the watchman house, I cried all the way home. I remember waking up crying a couple weeks before, sensing what was coming. God has given me the gift of prophecy; and at times that gift was a little frightening, to be honest, but this was just a warning to prepare myself. It's as if God was saying, "Hey, you got this. Everything will be ok; just look to me, and things will be better." The human inclination to fix everything kicks in when you have a special needs child. God was reminding me that you can't fix everything. Don't we hate hearing it is what it is, but maybe that is what it is, right?

When I finally reached the office the next morning, after dropping Jordan off at Mayes, I was told he was doing fine, and they had given him a bowl of ice cream to ease things the night before. Oh, how my heart ached for him; and now, to be honest at times, wanting a child to be typical who is atypical changes your world. It is like planning to go to Hawaii, but your plane stops in Iceland instead. You weren't expecting to go there but since you're there, you might as well make the best of it. *But how?* you ask yourself. This is tough. I ministered to myself, saying, "Everything will be ok; just keep your faith and keep your eyes on Jesus!"

How will my husband do with this? From my perspective, he was having a hard time with it, but he always said I took it much harder. My daughter was in seventh grade at the time, but how was this affecting her? What could I do or not do to help her through this? We adopted a little dog name Klaus not long after we left Jordan at Mayes. Maddi had always played with Jordan, loving him just as he was, not trying too hard to change him. I guess it was the parents who struggled to fix it.

When Jordan was first diagnosed, I put Maddi in a local Christian school, East Texas Christian school in Texas. The school is no longer there but what a blessing it was to Maddi and I, with all the speech therapy and ABA therapy (applied behavioral therapy) for Jordan that would ultimately take time away from my daughter. Then God made a way where there was no way. The Christian school and grandparents and cousins stepped up to the plate. They definitely made all the difference in filling in the gaps.

One of Jordan's counselors at his elementary helped by saying this, as parents, we do the best we can at the time. We look back to know that at the time, we made the best decision we knew how. I had called her at a time when I was trying to beat myself up for not getting help sooner. As I would come to discover, many children are diagnosed much later than my son was at three years old. I was told his brain was still pliable and we began our race against time.

I am now fifty-six ,and my husband is fifty-seven, and I look back thinking where did all this time go. We were so busy and caught up in our roles as parents, our careers as a scientist and a teacher, that we barely had time for each other. The clock kept ticking. I met a couple who had a son with autism, who were a scientist and a nurse. This couple had the child who pulled his permanent front teeth out in a fit of rage. How these parents must have suffered. Yes, God was answering our prayers, but now I had to help this couple see that Mayes would be a good option for them as well. Their son needed even more help than Jordan in a lot of ways.

Yes, as a child, my son had banged his head against our bar, had banged his head against metal poles at school. This was so traumatizing enough to us. Self-injurious behavior has to be the worse. I called an ambulance once because my son was so upset one morning, about what I'm not sure.

While getting ready for school one day, he banged his head against large stones on our fireplace. It was heart wrenching to know my son was upset and could not express his anger or sadness about whatever it was bothering him. He spit his medicine out that morning, also all over the floor. I don't think he liked school or maybe the kids were being mean to him. That day I needed to get to work, my husband also, my daughter to school. Madison didn't understand either what was happening with her brother.

One time, she had brought a friend over from the Christian school one day to play. Jordan was in the room playing with them, or so I thought. Then I heard the little girl running around in circles, calling my son the "r" word. How I hate that word. Well, the little girl was admonished and sent on her way, and this became a teaching moment for my daughter on how to choose our friends. The devil goes to Christian schools and churches too. Oh how I prayed for my son, oh how I prayed for my daughter, my husband and I. What about my marriage, how was this affecting my marriage? My husband began to travel and stay away from home as much as possible it seemed. This became a contention between us. I cried out to Jesus, "Help us, Lord Jesus. Bless our marriage, protect our marriage."

I can honestly say now looking back that I took everything that happened with my children way too hard. My earthly dad, Maurice, had warned me not to do this! It was so hard. I had anxiety then, but just didn't know to what extent. My son was seeing a psychiatrist, "Dr. Cupcakes," at the time. Yes, that was her nickname. Kids loved her. After my son knocked all the windows out of my house with an umbrella and put holes in almost every wall, broke my antique clock on the mantle my grandparent had given me, I broke down in tears and made an appointment to see Dr. Cupcakes for myself. She diagnosed me with anxiety disorder or GAD (generalized anxiety disorder) I had been struggling with this ever since I could remember. Maybe now, I would get some help with this sadness. I know where my true help comes from though; my help comes from the Lord!

I believe in miracles and that medicine would just be another tool in my toolbox. Untreated anxiety drives you and your family bananas (literally). I did not know, but I know now that we all have issues; but to my amazement, I did not know that I also had undiagnosed dyslexia at an early age. Thank you Jesus for my godly mother, who read to me every night and corrected my handwriting when I reversed letters. This was a sure sign of dyslexia but back in the early seventies, when I was learning to read and write, there were no dyslexia teachers.

All my memories from childhood rushed back when I got to college and decided to take a shorthand class. If you don't know what shorthand is, look it up. It is a dead art, no longer needed due to the rising artificial intelligence in play. In 1983, I began taking college courses as an eighteen-year old. I decided to major in business. So, of course, shorthand would be one of my first summer courses in the summer of 1983. I started out thinking I would be a communications major. But that didn't pan out, seeing that I changed majors, along with the boyfriend I was dating at the time.

My brother Chad had commented once on how I changed what music I liked depending on the guy I was dating at the time. I didn't meet my husband until 1987. By this time, he had graduated Lamar University and he had lost his dad to a brain aneurysm at the young age of fifty-one. So, my children did not know his dad, and neither did I. I'm sure that was part of the reason my husband and mother-in-law cried at our wedding. The years flew by as we married in 1989, had our first child, who is now a nurse practitioner about to graduate from Texas Women's University this August with her masters. We will have a great big party with friends and family when this great feat occurs.

I once read how having a sibling with special needs can go either of two ways. All I can say now is thank you to my savior Jesus for Maddi's life. It went the right way, God's way. God is ordering our steps now; I am sure of it. In the struggles and trials of life, have you running to Christ or away from Christ? Thankfully, my children and I have run toward Him with open arms. The love He has for each of us is so overwhelming, but how can it be?

My Bible study group on Facebook is called "Faith Gathers," and this week we talked about how we finish our races. We talked about how keeping our faith through every trial and blessing shows who we are and what we do. We are the influencers of the Christian faith, and how we react to our problems and blessings tell a lot about our character and God's character. As Christians, it should tell of Jesus's character because we are not our own; we are His tools. We were bought with a very high price. Jesus paid it all, and He overcame the world, so we can rest assured He has our backs through it all. To God should be the glory for it all.

CPSIA information can be obtained
at www.ICGtesting.com
Printed in the USA
BVHW081324310821
615689BV00002B/180